MEAL PREP GUIDE FOR WEIGHT LOSS

Plan and savor: Healthy and delicious recipes for beginners

SHELLEY WEBSTER

TABLE OF CONTENTS

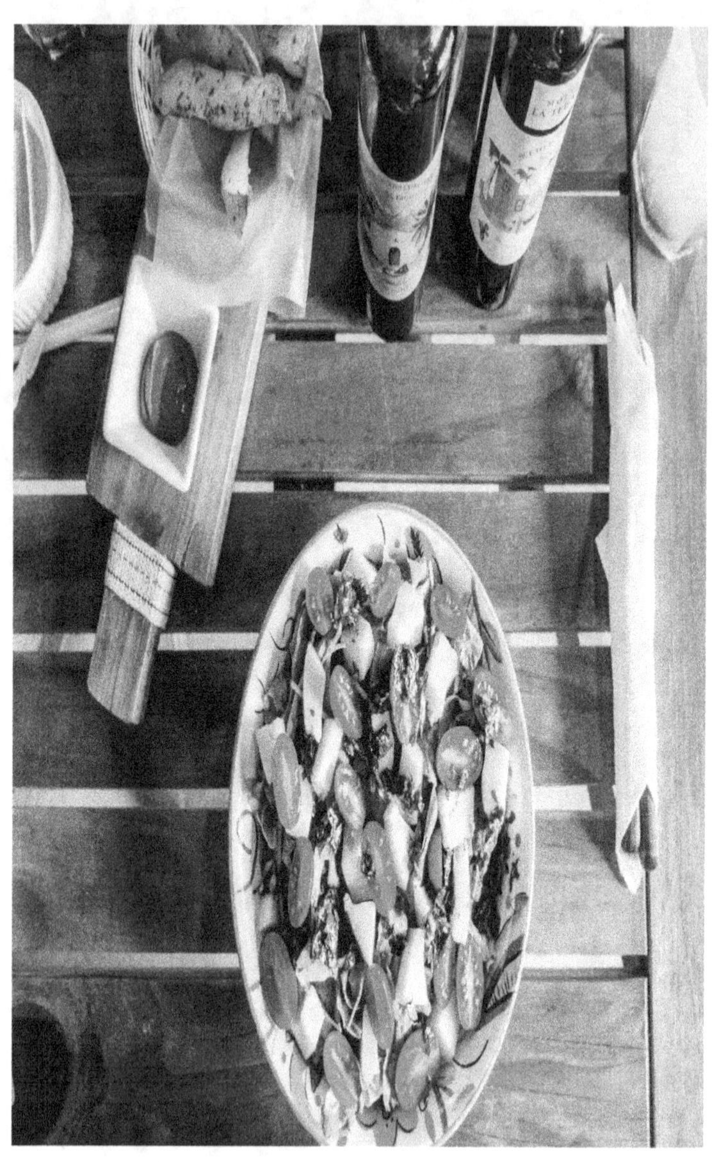

INTRODUCTION

Welcome to the journey towards a healthier, happier you! If you've decided to embark on the path to weight loss and overall well-being, you've taken a significant step towards a positive transformation. This meal prep guide is designed to be your trusted companion on this journey, offering you the knowledge, tools, and delicious recipes to help you achieve your weight loss goals while savoring every bite along the way.

In today's fast-paced world, making healthier food choices can often feel like a daunting task. We understand the challenges you may face—juggling work, family, and other responsibilities can leave little time for mindful eating. That's where meal prep comes in as your secret weapon. By planning and preparing your meals in advance, you regain control over what you eat, ensure balanced nutrition, and eliminate the guesswork that often leads to unhealthy choices.

But this isn't just another meal prep guide; it's a comprehensive resource tailored specifically to your weight loss journey. We'll walk you through the essential steps of meal planning, teach you how to shop smart, and provide you with a treasure trove of healthy and delicious recipes. Whether you're a seasoned meal prepper or a complete novice, you'll find valuable insights and inspiration within these pages.

Remember, achieving and maintaining a healthy weight isn't just about temporary changes. It's about building sustainable habits that become a natural part of your life. It's about feeling energized, confident, and vibrant every day. So, as you embark on this adventure, keep in mind that it's not just about losing weight; it's about gaining a healthier and happier you

Are you ready to take the first step? Let's dive in and start your meal prep journey towards a healthier, more vibrant future!

The Importance of Meal Prep for Weight Loss

Embarking on a weight loss journey is a significant commitment, and it often requires more than just good intentions. Meal prep, the process of planning, preparing, and portioning your meals in advance, can be a game-changer on your path to weight loss success. Here's why it's so crucial:

1. **Portion Control:** One of the leading causes of weight gain is overeating, and it's easy to fall into this trap when you're not mindful of your portions. Meal prep allows you to control portion sizes, ensuring you consume the right amount of calories to support your weight loss goals.

2. **Consistency:** Consistency is key in weight loss. By having pre-prepared, healthy meals on hand, you're less likely to succumb to unhealthy, convenient options when you're hungry and in a rush. Meal prep keeps you on track.

3. **Balanced Nutrition:** Achieving and maintaining a healthy weight isn't just about cutting calories. It's also about getting the right nutrients. With meal prep, you can carefully plan balanced meals that provide the vitamins, minerals, and macronutrients your body needs.

4. **Reduction of Temptation:** When you've already prepared your meals, you're less likely to give in to unhealthy cravings or fast food temptations. You've got a nutritious option ready to go, making it easier to stick to your plan.

5. **Time and Stress Management:** We all live busy lives, and finding time to cook healthy meals every day can be a significant challenge. Meal prep saves your time during the week and reduces the stress of figuring out what to eat each day.

6. **Financial Savings:** Eating out or ordering takeout regularly can strain your budget. Meal prepping can help you save money by buying ingredients in bulk and avoiding expensive restaurant meals.

7. **Long-Term Success:** Weight loss isn't just about shedding pounds temporarily. It's about creating lasting, healthy habits. Meal prep teaches you to make intentional food choices and encourages mindful eating, setting you up for long-term success.

8. **Empowerment:** Meal prep puts you in control of your nutrition. You decide what goes into your meals, ensuring that they align with your dietary preferences and restrictions.

In this guide, we'll delve into the art of meal prep, providing you with the knowledge, tools, and delicious recipes you need to make it an integral part of your weight loss journey. With dedication and a well-organized meal prep routine, you can achieve your weight loss goals while enjoying tasty, nutritious meals.

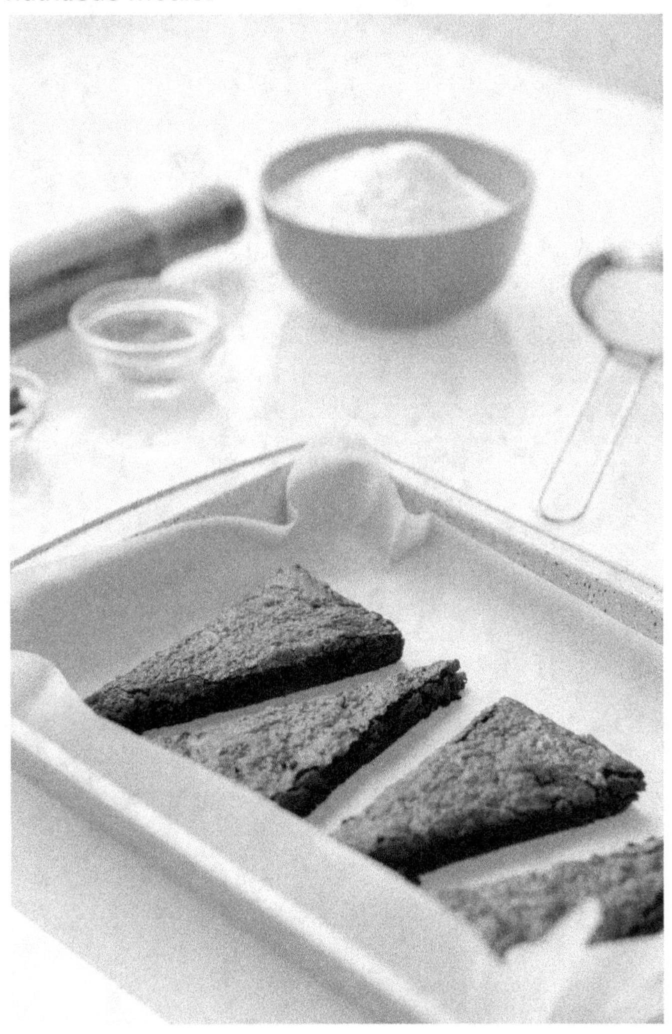

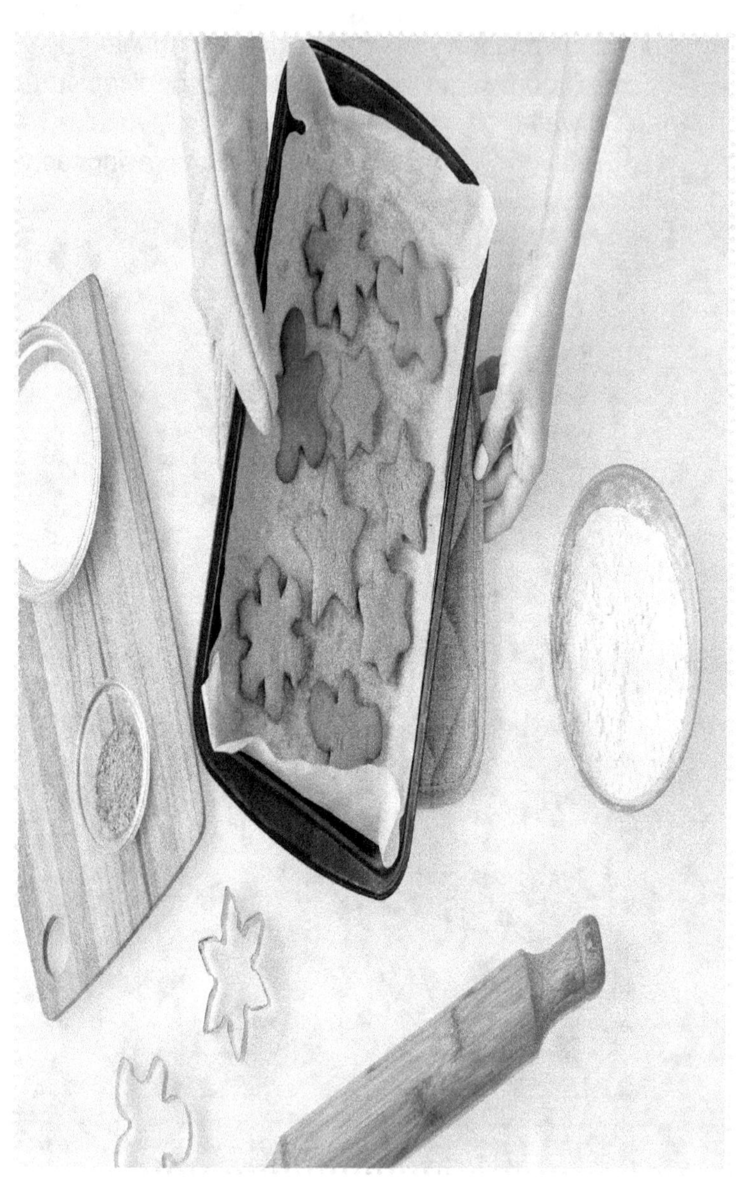

How This Guide Can Help You

Certainly! Here's a section on "How This Guide Can Help You" for your meal prep guide:

Congratulations on taking the first step toward your weight loss goals! We understand that embarking on a journey to lose weight and improve your health can be both exciting and challenging. This comprehensive meal prep guide is designed to be your reliable companion throughout this transformative process. Here's how it can assist you on your path to success:

1. **Education and Insight:** This guide provides you with valuable knowledge about meal prep, nutrition, and weight loss. You'll learn the science behind healthy eating and discover practical tips and strategies to make informed choices.

2. **Meal Planning Made Simple:** We'll walk you through the process of creating personalized meal plans tailored to your calorie and nutrients. Say goodbye to confusion and hello to organized, balanced meals.

3. **Delicious and Nutritious Recipes:** Inside these pages, you'll find a treasure trove of mouthwatering recipes designed to tantalize your taste buds while supporting your weight loss goals.

From breakfast to dinner and even desserts, we've got you covered.

4. **Time and Effort Savings:** We understand that your time is precious. With our meal prep strategies, you'll save time in the kitchen during the week, allowing you to focus on other important aspects of your life.

5. **Empowerment:** This guide aims to empower you with knowledge and skills to take control of your eating habits. You'll learn to make food choices that align with your goals and preferences.

6. **Consistency and Accountability:** Meal prep fosters consistency, making it easier to stick to your weight loss plan. By having healthy meals readily available, you'll be less likely to deviate from your goals.

7. **Support and Encouragement:** I'mWe're here to support you every step of the way. Whether you're facing challenges, seeking motivation, or simply looking for guidance, this guide is your trusted resource.

8. **Sustainability:** Weight loss isn't just about reaching a number on the scale; it's about adopting a healthier, more sustainable lifestyle. We'll help you transition from short-term changes to long-term habits that promote well-being.

By using this guide as your roadmap, you're not only setting yourself up for weight loss success but also for a brighter, healthier future. Remember, you have the power to take charge of your nutrition and transform your life. Let's begin this exciting journey together!

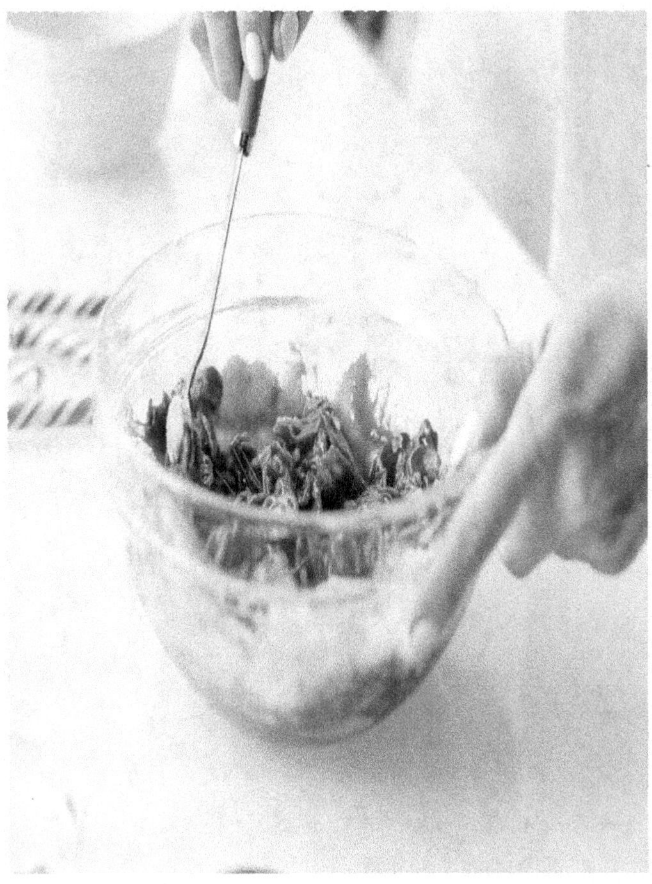

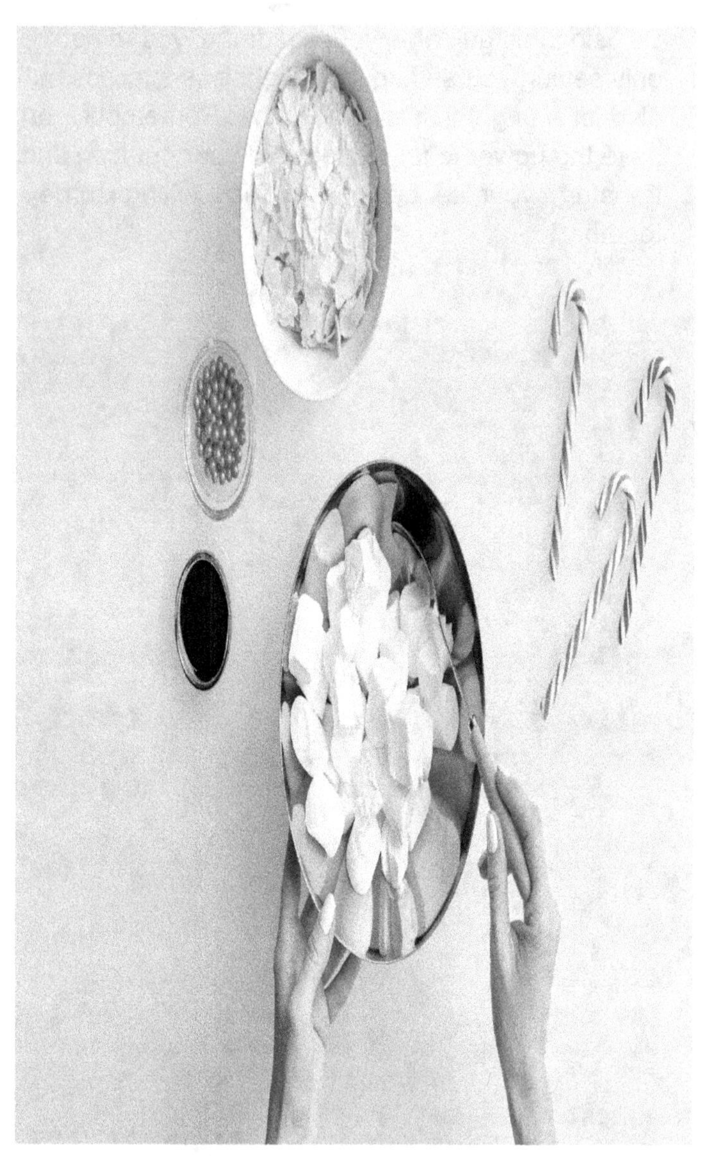

CHAPTER ONE

Getting Started

Certainly! Here's a section on "Getting Started" for your meal prep guide:

Congratulations on taking the first step towards a healthier you! Embarking on a weight loss journey is an empowering decision, and the journey begins with a solid foundation. In this section, we'll guide you through the essential steps to set you up for success.

1. Setting Your Weight Loss Goals:

Before you dive into meal prep, it's crucial to define your weight loss goals. Ask yourself:

- How much weight do you want to lose?
- What's your target timeframe for achieving your goals?
- Are there specific health or fitness milestones you want to reach?

Having clear, realistic goals will give you a sense of purpose and help you stay motivated throughout your journey.

2. Assessing Your Current Eating Habits:

Understanding your current eating patterns is key to making positive changes. Take some time to:

- Keep a food diary for a few days to track what you eat and when.
- Identify any unhealthy eating habits or triggers (e.g., emotional eating, late-night snacking).
- Recognize foods that may be contributing to weight gain or hindering your progress.

This self-assessment will help you pinpoint areas that need improvement and give you insights into your eating behaviors.

3. Gathering the Right Meal Prep Tools:

To make meal prep efficient and enjoyable, you'll need the right tools. Start by ensuring you have:

- **Storage Containers:** Invest in a variety of containers in different sizes to store your prepared meals.
- **Kitchen Essentials:** Stock your kitchen with basic cooking utensils, pots, pans, and sharp knives.
- **Meal Planning Tools:** Consider using apps or templates to create meal plans and shopping lists.

By having these tools at your disposal, you'll be well-prepared for your meal prep journey. Remember, getting started is often the most challenging part. However, by setting clear goals, understanding your current habits, and equipping yourself with the right tools, you're laying a solid foundation for success. In the following sections, we'll dive deeper into the world of meal planning, grocery shopping, and the art of meal prep, all of which will play pivotal roles in your weight loss journey.

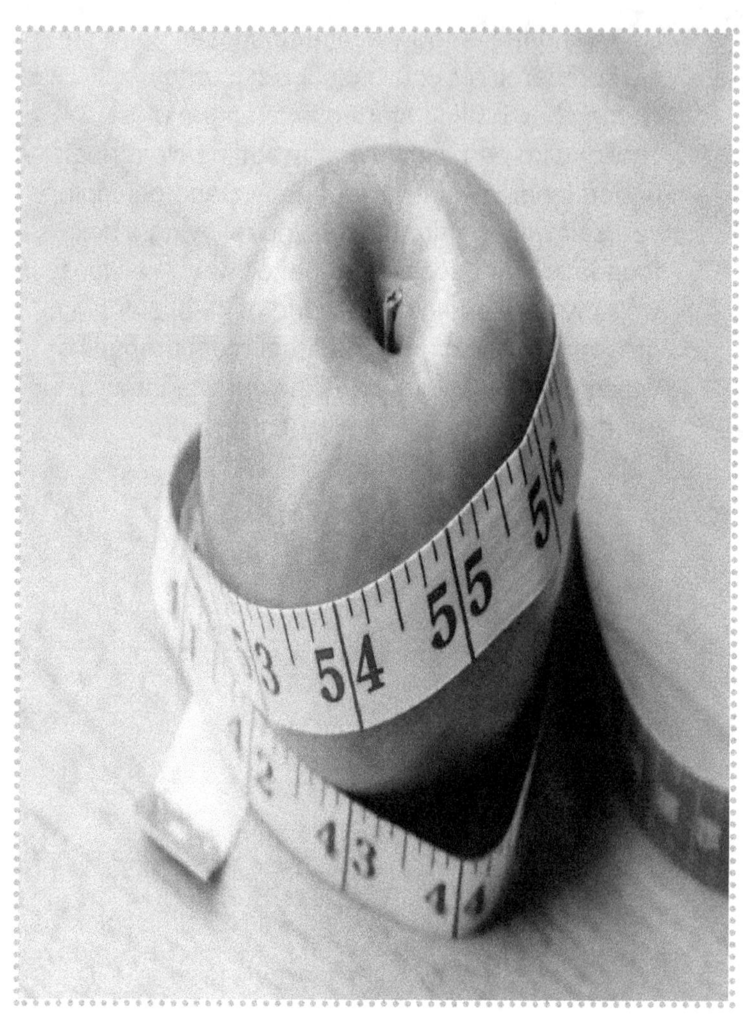

CHAPTER TWO

Planning Your Meals

Certainly! Here's a section on "Planning Your Meals" for your meal prep guide:

Effective meal planning is the cornerstone of successful meal prep and weight loss. It's the roadmap that ensures you're consuming the right foods in the right amounts to achieve your goals. In this section, we'll guide you through the process of creating a meal plan that's tailored to your needs.

1. Creating a Balanced Meal Plan:

A balanced meal plan is one that provides your body with the essential nutrients it needs to thrive while helping you reach your weight loss goals. Here's how to do it:

Divide Your Plate: Aim to fill half your plate with vegetables, one-quarter with lean protein (e.g., chicken, fish, tofu), and one-quarter with complex carbohydrates (e.g., brown rice, quinoa).

Incorporate Variety: Ensure your meal plan includes a wide range of foods to prevent boredom and provide a diverse array of nutrients.

Control Portion Sizes: Be mindful of portion sizes to manage your calorie intake. Use measuring cups or a food scale if needed.

2. Calculating Calorie and Macronutrient Needs:

The number of calories and the balance of macronutrients (protein, carbohydrates, and fats) you need can vary based on factors like your age, gender, activity level, and weight loss goals. Here's how to calculate your requirements:

- **Calories:** Use an online calculator or consult a healthcare professional to determine your daily calorie needs for weight loss.

- **Macronutrients:** Once you have your calorie target, decide on your macronutrient ratio. A common guideline is 40% carbohydrates, 30% protein, and 30% fat, but this can vary based on individual preferences and dietary restrictions.

3. Tips for Successful Meal Planning:

To make meal planning easier and more effective, consider the following tips:

Batch Cooking: Plan to cook larger batches of food that you can use for multiple meals. This saves time and ensures you have healthy options readily available.

Pre-Portion Snacks: Prepare snack-sized portions of healthy options like nuts, fruits, or yogurt to avoid mindless munching on high-calorie snacks.

Plan for Special Occasions: If you know you have a special event or meal out planned, adjust your meal plan accordingly to accommodate these occasions while staying within your overall calorie goals.

Stay Flexible: Your meal plan is a guide, not a strict rule. Be flexible and open to adjustments as needed. Life can be unpredictable, and it's essential to adapt your plan when necessary.

Creating a well-thought-out meal plan not only supports your weight loss goals but also makes meal prep more efficient. It's like having a blueprint for your healthy eating journey. In the upcoming sections, we'll explore practical strategies for grocery shopping, meal prep, and making most of your planned meals. Let's continue on this path to a healthier lifestyle!

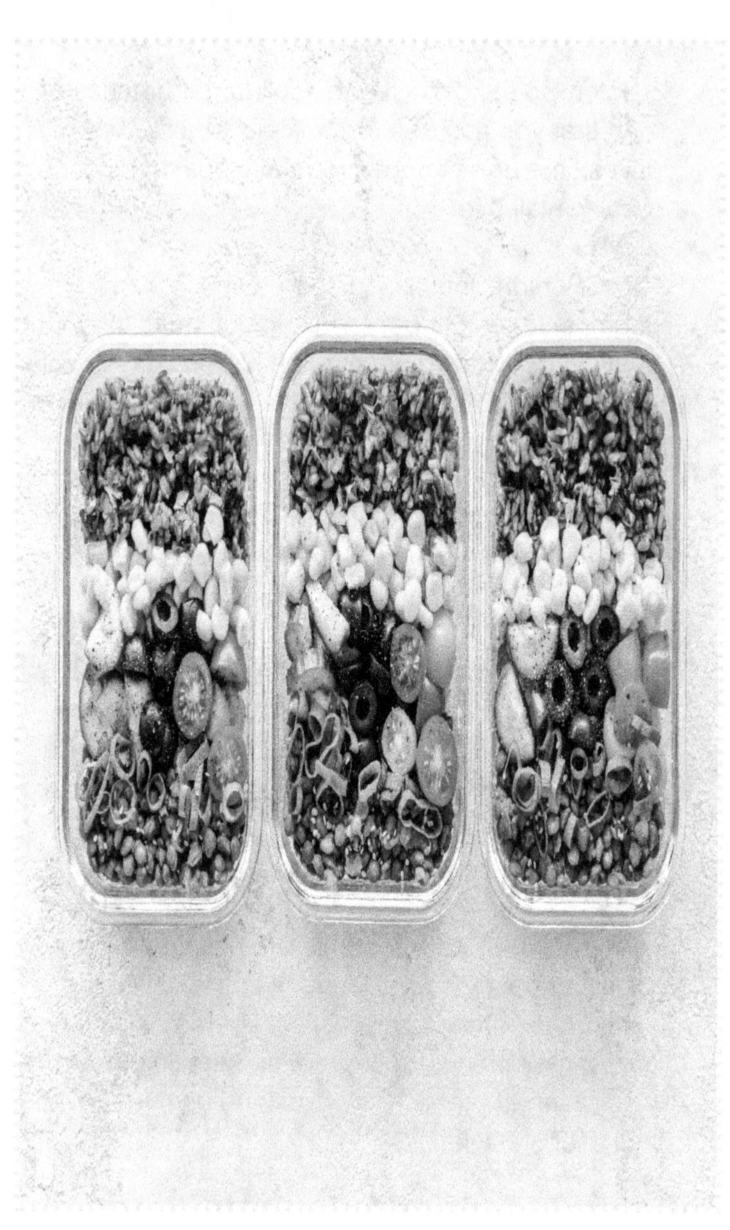

CHAPTER THREE

Shopping Smart

Absolutely! Here's a section on "Shopping Smart" for your meal prep guide:

The success of your meal prep and weight loss journey often begins at the grocery store. Smart and strategic shopping can set the stage for healthier eating throughout the week. In this section, we'll explore how to make informed choices, save money, and select the best ingredients for your meals.

1. Building a Weight Loss Grocery List:

Before you hit the supermarket, it's essential to have a well-thought-out grocery list. Here's how to create one:

- **Plan Your Meals:** Refer to your meal plan and identify the ingredients you need for the week's recipes.

- **Organize Your List:** Group items by category (e.g., produce, dairy, protein) to streamline your shopping trip.

- **Stick to the List:** Avoid impulsive purchases by adhering to your list. If it's not on the list, reconsider whether you truly need it.

2. Understanding Food Labels:

Reading food labels is a crucial skill when shopping for weight loss. Pay attention to:

- **Calories:** Check the calorie content per serving to ensure it aligns with your meal plan.

- **Portion Sizes:** Be aware of the number of servings in a package, as this can affect calorie intake.

- **Nutrient Content:** Look for products with lower saturated fats, added sugars, and sodium. Opt for higher fiber and protein options.

- **Ingredients List:** Familiarize yourself with the ingredients used. Avoid products with a long list of additives and preservatives.

3. Budget-Friendly Shopping Strategies:

Eating healthily doesn't have to break the bank. Consider these tips to save money while shopping:

- **Buy in Bulk:** Purchase non-perishable items like grains, beans, and canned goods in bulk to reduce the cost per serving.

- **Use Coupons and Sales:** Take advantage of discounts, coupons, and sales to save on items you regularly use.

- **Choose Seasonal Produce:** Seasonal fruits and vegetables are often more affordable and fresher.

- **Compare Prices:** Compare prices across different brands and store brands to find the best deals.

4. Healthy Shopping Habits:

Maintain healthy shopping habits to stay on track:

Shop the Perimeter: The perimeter of the store typically contains fresh produce, protein, and dairy. Focus on these areas for healthier options.

Don't Shop Hungry: Eat a small, balanced meal or snack before shopping to avoid impulse purchases of unhealthy items.

Avoid Aisles with Temptations: If certain aisles or sections of the store are filled with items that tempt you, consider avoiding them altogether.

Stay Mindful: Keep your health and weight loss goals in mind as you shop. Make conscious choices that align with your objectives.

Smart shopping is a vital skill for successful meal prep and weight loss. By planning ahead, making informed choices, and staying mindful of your goals, you can fill your cart with nutritious ingredients that support your journey to a healthier you. In the upcoming sections, we'll delve into the practical aspects of meal prep, ensuring that your smart shopping translates into delicious and nutritious meals.

CHAPTER FOUR

Healthy Breakfast Recipes

Certainly! Here's a section on "Healthy Breakfast Recipes" for your meal prep guide:

They say that breakfast is the most important meal of the day, and when you're on a weight loss journey, it's essential to start your day right. These healthy and delicious breakfast recipes will not only kickstart your morning but also keep you satisfied until your next meal.

1. Overnight Oats

Ingredients:
- 1/2 cup rolled oats
- 1/2 cup unsweetened almond milk (or your choice of milk)
- 1/4 cup Greek yogurt
- 1 tablespoon chia seeds
- 1/2 teaspoon honey or maple syrup
- Fresh berries and sliced almonds for topping

Instructions:
1. In a mason jar or airtight container, combine oats, almond milk, Greek yogurt, chia seeds, and honey or maple syrup.

2. Stir well, seal, and refrigerate overnight.
3. In the morning, top with fresh berries and sliced almonds before serving.

2. Veggie and Egg Breakfast Muffins

Ingredients:
- 6 large eggs
- 1/2 cup diced bell peppers
- 1/2 cup diced spinach
- 1/4 cup diced tomatoes
- 1/4 cup diced onions
- Salt and pepper to taste
- Optional: grated cheese

Instructions:
1. Preheat your oven to 350°F (175°C) and grease a muffin tin.
2. In a bowl, whisk together the eggs, salt, and pepper.
3. Divide the diced vegetables evenly into each muffin cup.
4. Pour the egg mixture over the veggies, filling each cup about 2/3 full.
5. If desired, sprinkle with grated cheese.
6. Bake for 20-25 minutes until the eggs are set and lightly browned.
7. Allow to cool before removing from the muffin tin.

3. Greek Yogurt Parfait

Ingredients:
- 1 cup Greek yogurt
- 1/2 cup mixed berries (e.g., strawberries, blueberries)
- 1/4 cup granola
- Honey for drizzling (optional)

Instructions:
1. In a glass or bowl, layer Greek yogurt, mixed berries, and granola.
2. Repeat the layers.
3. Drizzle with honey if desired.
4. Enjoy immediately or seal for a grab-and-go breakfast.

These breakfast recipes are not only nutritious but also easy to prepare in advance for your busy mornings. They provide the energy and nutrients you need to kickstart your day on the right foot and keep you on track with your weight loss goals. In the following sections, we'll explore equally enticing lunch and dinner recipes, making your weight loss journey both tasty and satisfying.

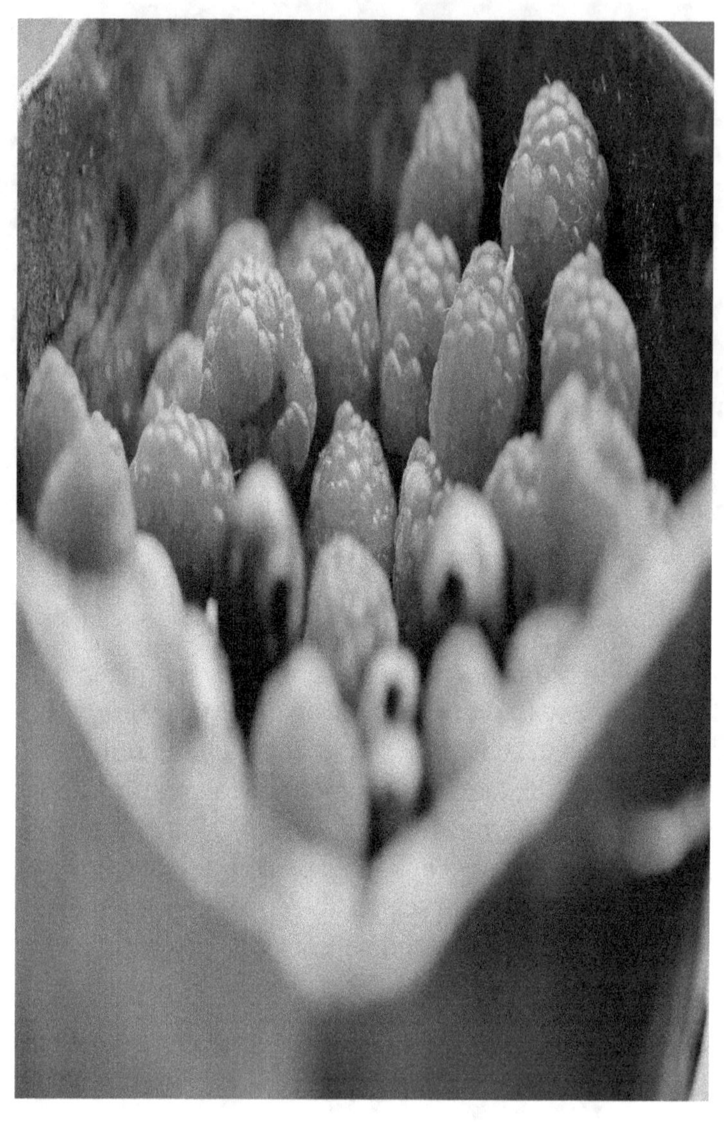

CHAPTER FIVE

Wholesome Lunch Ideas

Certainly! Here's a section on "Wholesome Lunch Ideas" for your meal prep guide:

Lunch is an important opportunity to refuel and stay energized throughout the day. These wholesome lunch ideas are not only delicious but also designed to keep you satisfied while supporting your weight loss goals.

1. Grilled Chicken Salad with Balsamic Vinaigrette

Ingredients:
- Grilled chicken breast strips
- Mixed greens (e.g., spinach, arugula, kale)
- Cherry tomatoes, halved
- Cucumber slices
- Red onion, thinly sliced
- Avocado slices
- Balsamic vinaigrette dressing (choose a light or low-fat version)

Instructions:

1. Toss the mixed greens with cherry tomatoes,
cucumber slices, red onion, and avocado slices.
2. Top the salad with grilled chicken breast strips.
3. Drizzle with balsamic vinaigrette dressing.

2. Quinoa and Black Bean Bowl

Ingredients:
- Cooked quinoa
- Black beans, drained and rinsed
- Roasted or steamed vegetables (e.g., bell
peppers, broccoli, carrots)
- Salsa or a homemade yogurt-based dressing
- Fresh cilantro for garnish

Instructions:
1. In a bowl, combine cooked quinoa, black beans,
and roasted or steamed vegetables.
2. Drizzle with salsa or a yogurt-based dressing for
added flavor.
3. Garnish with fresh cilantro.

3. Turkey and Avocado Wrap

Ingredients:
- Whole-grain tortilla or wrap
- Sliced turkey breast (or a vegetarian alternative)

- Sliced avocado
- Spinach leaves
- Sliced red bell pepper
- Hummus or light mayo (optional)

Instructions:
1. Lay the whole-grain tortilla flat.
2. Spread a thin layer of hummus or light mayo
(optional) on the tortilla.
3. Layer with sliced turkey, avocado, spinach
leaves, and red bell pepper.
4. Roll up the tortilla, slice in half, and secure with
toothpicks.

4. Lentil and Vegetable Soup

Ingredients:
- Cooked lentils
- Mixed vegetables (e.g., carrots, celery, zucchini)
- Low-sodium vegetable broth
- Herbs and spices (e.g., thyme, oregano, paprika)
- Salt and pepper to taste

Instructions:
1. In a pot, combine cooked lentils, mixed
vegetables, and vegetable broth.
2. Season with your choice of herbs and spices.
3. Simmer until the vegetables are tender and the
flavors meld together.

These wholesome lunch ideas are not only satisfying but also provide the nutrients and energy you need to power through your day. They can be wrapped in advance, making it convenient to stick to your weight loss plan on busy days. In the following sections, we'll explore delightful dinner recipes and strategies to maintain your weight loss momentum. Enjoy your wholesome lunches!

CHAPTER SIX

Prepping for Success

Certainly! Here's a section on "Prepping for Success" for your meal prep guide:

Meal prep is the secret to stay on track with your weight loss goals while enjoying nutritious and delicious meals. This section will guide you through essential steps to ensure you are well-prepared for your meal prep journey.

1. Time-Saving Meal Prep Tips:

Efficiency is key when it comes to meal prep. Consider these time-saving tips:

- **Plan Ahead:** Set aside a specific day or time each week for meal prep. Consistency is your ally.

- **Use Multi-Tasking Techniques:** Cook multiple components simultaneously to save time. For example, while roasting vegetables, you can also cook a batch of grains or proteins.

- **Invest in Helpful Tools:** Equip your kitchen with time-saving tools like a food processor for chopping, a slow cooker for easy one-pot meals, and a good set of knives for efficient slicing and dicing.

2. Batch Cooking Techniques:

Batch cooking is the heart of meal prep. Here's how to master it:

- **Cook in Bulk:** Prepare larger quantities of staple ingredients like brown rice, quinoa, or lean proteins that you can use for multiple meals.

- **Portion Control:** Divide cooked food into meal-sized portions, making it easy to grab and go during the week.

- **Freeze for Later:** Some dishes freeze well, allowing you to prepare meals weeks in advance. Soups, stews, and casseroles are excellent candidates for freezing.

3. Organizing Your Kitchen for Efficiency:

An organized kitchen is your secret weapon for successful meal prep:

- **Clear the Clutter:** Declutter your kitchen counters and cabinets to create more workspace.

- **Organize Your Pantry:** Group similar items together in your pantry and label containers for easy access.

- **Designate a Meal Prep Zone:** Dedicate a specific area of your kitchen to meal prep. This keeps all your tools and ingredients in one place.

4. Meal Prep Safety:

Safety is paramount during meal prep:

- **Practice Safe Food Handling:** Wash your hands, utensils, and cutting boards thoroughly. Keep raw and cooked foods separate to prevent cross-contamination.

- **Proper Storage:** Use airtight containers to store prepped ingredients and meals. Refrigerate or freeze promptly to maintain freshness.

- **Label and Date:** Label containers with the date of preparation to keep track of freshness.

Prepping for success means setting yourself up for an easier, healthier, and more enjoyable week ahead. With efficient techniques, a well-organized kitchen, and a focus on safety, you'll find that meal prep becomes a natural part of your routine. In the upcoming sections, we'll dive into the heart of meal prep—creating delicious and nutritious meals that support your weight loss goals. Let's continue on this journey to a healthier you!

CHAPTER SEVEN

Flavorful Dinner Recipes**

Certainly! Here's a section on "Flavorful Dinner Recipes" for your meal prep guide:

Dinner is a time to unwind and savor a delicious meal, even when you're on a weight loss journey. These flavorful dinner recipes are not only nutritious but also designed to satisfy your taste buds.

1. Baked Salmon with Lemon and Dill

Ingredients:
- Salmon fillets
- Fresh lemon slices
- Fresh dill sprigs
- Olive oil
- Salt and pepper to taste

Instructions:
1. Preheat your oven to 375°F (190°C).
2. Place salmon fillets on a baking sheet lined with parchment paper.
3. Drizzle with olive oil and season with salt and pepper.

4. Top each filet with fresh lemon slices and dill sprigs.
5. Bake for 15-20 minutes or until the salmon flakes easily with a fork.

2. Veggie Stir-Fry with Tofu

Ingredients:
- Firm tofu, cubed
- Mixed stir-fry vegetables (e.g., broccoli, bell peppers, snap peas)
- Low-sodium soy sauce or teriyaki sauce
- Minced garlic and ginger
- Cooked brown rice or quinoa

Instructions:
1. In a pan or wok, sauté cubed tofu until lightly browned. Remove from the pan.
2. In the same pan, add minced garlic and ginger, followed by the mixed vegetables.
3. Stir-fry until the vegetables are tender-crisp.
4. Return the tofu to the pan and drizzle with low-sodium soy sauce or teriyaki sauce.
5. Serve over cooked brown rice or quinoa.

3. Spaghetti Squash with Tomato and Basil

Ingredients:
- Spaghetti squash
- Fresh tomatoes, diced
- Fresh basil leaves, chopped
- Garlic, minced
- Olive oil
- Salt and pepper to taste
- Grated Parmesan cheese (optional)

Instructions:
1. Preheat your oven to 375°F (190°C).
2. Cut the spaghetti squash in half lengthwise and scoop out the seeds.
3. Drizzle olive oil over the cut sides, and season with salt and pepper.
4. Place the squash halves cut-side down on a baking sheet and roast for about 45 minutes, or until the flesh can be easily shredded with a fork.
5. In a pan, sauté minced garlic until fragrant, then add diced tomatoes and fresh basil. Cook until the tomatoes soften.
6. Use a fork to shred the cooked spaghetti squash into "noodles."
7. Top the squash noodles with tomato and basil mixture.
8. Optionally, sprinkle with grated Parmesan cheese.

4. Grilled Chicken with Lemon and Herbs

Ingredients:
- Chicken breasts or thighs
- Fresh lemon juice
- Fresh herbs (e.g., rosemary, thyme, oregano)
- Olive oil
- Salt and pepper to taste

Instructions:
1. Preheat your grill to medium-high heat.
2. In a bowl, mix fresh lemon juice, olive oil, chopped herbs, salt, and pepper.
3. Brush the mixture onto the chicken.
4. Grill the chicken until it's cooked through, with grill marks and a slightly charred exterior.

These flavorful dinner recipes are designed to keep your taste buds delighted while supporting your weight loss goals. They can be prepared in advance and enjoyed as part of your meal prep routine. In the following sections, we'll discuss snacks, desserts, and long-term strategies to maintain your healthy eating habits. Enjoy your flavorful dinners!

CHAPTER EIGHT

Snack Smart

Certainly! Here's a section on "Snack Smart" for your meal prep guide:

Snacking can be a part of a balanced diet, even during a weight loss journey. However, making smart snack choices is essential. These snack ideas are both nutritious and satisfying, helping you stay on track while curbing cravings.

1. Greek Yogurt and Berries

Ingredients:
- Greek yogurt (unsweetened)
- Fresh or frozen berries (e.g., strawberries, blueberries)

Instructions:
- Simply top a bowl of Greek yogurt with a handful of fresh or frozen berries for a creamy and antioxidant-rich snack.

2. Veggie Sticks with Hummus

Ingredients:
- Sliced cucumber, carrot, and bell pepper
- Hummus (choose a lower-fat variety)

Instructions:
- Pair your favorite veggies with a generous scoop of hummus for a crunchy and protein-packed snack.

3. Apple Slices with Almond Butter

Ingredients:
- Apple slices
- Almond butter (or your choice of nut butter)

Instructions:
- Spread almond butter onto apple slices for a sweet and satisfying snack that combines fiber and healthy fats.

4. Hard-Boiled Eggs

Ingredients:
- Hard-boiled eggs

Instructions:

- Hard-boiled eggs are a protein-rich snack that's easy to prepare in advance and keep in the fridge.

5. Air-Popped Popcorn

Ingredients:
- Air-popped popcorn (season lightly with herbs and spices)

Instructions:
- Popcorn can be a low-calorie and satisfying snack when prepared without excessive butter or oil.

6. Trail Mix

Ingredients:
- Nuts (e.g., almonds, walnuts)
- Seeds (e.g., pumpkin seeds, sunflower seeds)
- Dried fruits (e.g., raisins, apricots)

Instructions:
- Create your own trail mix with a balanced combination of nuts, seeds, and dried fruits. Portion control is key.

7. Cottage Cheese with Pineapple

Ingredients:
- Low-fat cottage cheese
- Pineapple chunks (fresh or canned in juice, not syrup)

Instructions:
- Top a serving of cottage cheese with pineapple chunks for a protein-packed and slightly sweet snack.

8. Sliced Bell Peppers with Guacamole

Ingredients:
- Sliced bell peppers (various colors)
- Guacamole (homemade or store-bought)

Instructions:
- Dip bell pepper slices into guacamole for a satisfying and vitamin-rich snack.

9. Greek Yogurt Parfait

Ingredients:
- Greek yogurt (unsweetened)
- Granola (choose a lower-sugar variety)
- Fresh berries

Instructions:

- Layer Greek yogurt, granola, and fresh berries to create a parfait that combines protein, fiber, and antioxidants.

10. Oatmeal with Banana

Ingredients:
- Plain oatmeal (cooked with water or milk)
- Sliced banana

Instructions:
- Top your oatmeal with sliced banana for a filling and naturally sweet snack.

Remember to practice portion control when snacking and stay mindful of your overall daily calorie intake. These smart snack ideas can help curb hunger and keep you energized throughout the day without derailing your weight loss efforts. In the following sections, we'll explore ways to enjoy dessert guilt-free and maintain your healthy eating habits long-term.

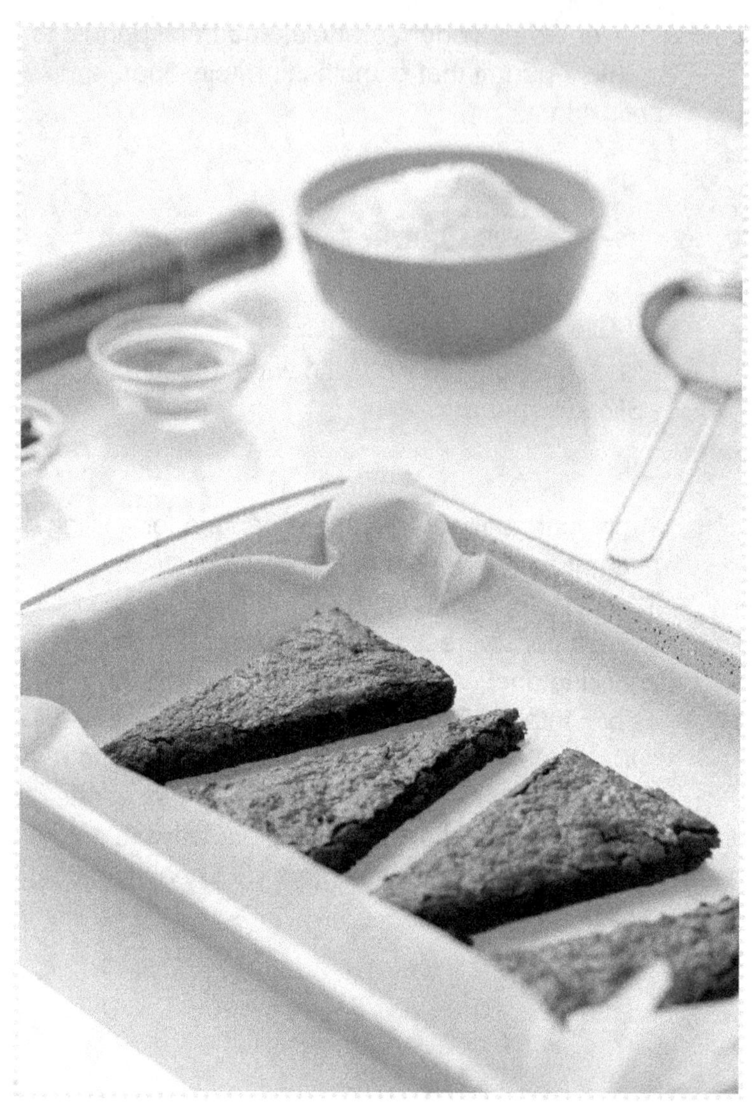

CHAPTER NINE

Desserts Without Guilt

Certainly! Here's a section on "Desserts Without Guilt" for your meal prep guide:

 Craving something sweet but want to stay on track with your weight loss goals? These dessert ideas are not only delicious but also guilt-free, allowing you to satisfy your sweet tooth without derailing your progress.

1. Chocolate Avocado Mousse

Ingredients:
- Ripe avocados
- Unsweetened cocoa powder
- Honey or maple syrup (for sweetness)
- A pinch of salt
- Vanilla extract

Instructions:
1. Blend ripe avocados, cocoa powder, honey or maple syrup, a pinch of salt, and a splash of vanilla extract until creamy.
2. Chill in the refrigerator for a few hours before serving.

2. Frozen Banana "Ice Cream"

Ingredients:
- Ripe bananas, sliced and frozen
- Optional add-ins: vanilla extract, cocoa powder, peanut butter

Instructions:
1. Blend frozen banana slices until smooth.
2. Add optional ingredients like vanilla extract, cocoa powder, or a spoonful of peanut butter for flavor.
3. Freeze briefly for a firmer texture or enjoy immediately for a soft-serve consistency.

3. Berry and Yogurt Parfait

Ingredients:
- Greek yogurt (unsweetened)
- Fresh berries (e.g., strawberries, blueberries, raspberries)
- A drizzle of honey (optional)
- Granola (choose a lower-sugar variety)

Instructions:
1. Layer Greek yogurt, fresh berries, and a drizzle of honey (if desired) in a glass or bowl.
2. Top with a sprinkle of granola for added crunch.

4. Chia Seed Pudding

Ingredients:
- Chia seeds
- Unsweetened almond milk (or your choice of milk)
- Vanilla extract
- A touch of honey or maple syrup (for sweetness)
- Fresh fruit for topping

Instructions:
1. Mix chia seeds, almond milk, vanilla extract, and a touch of honey or maple syrup in a jar or bowl.
2. Refrigerate for a few hours or overnight until the mixture thickens into a pudding-like consistency.
3. Top with fresh fruit before serving.

5. Fruit Salad with Mint

Ingredients:
- A variety of fresh fruits (e.g., watermelon, cantaloupe, kiwi, berries)
- Fresh mint leaves
- A squeeze of lime juice

Instructions:
1. Combine fresh fruits in a bowl.
2. Garnish with torn fresh mint leaves and a squeeze of lime juice for a refreshing dessert.

6. Baked Apple with Cinnamon

Ingredients:
- Apple, cored and sliced
- A sprinkle of cinnamon
- A drizzle of honey (optional)

Instructions:
1. Place apple slices on a baking sheet.
2. Sprinkle with cinnamon and drizzle with honey (if desired).
3. Bake until tender and slightly caramelized.

These guilt-free dessert ideas allow you to indulge in something sweet while staying aligned with your weight loss goals. They emphasize natural sweetness and whole ingredients, making them a healthier choice compared to traditional desserts. In the following sections, we'll discuss strategies for maintaining your healthy eating habits in the long run.

CHAPTER TEN

Weekly Meal Prep Plans

Certainly! Here's a section on "Weekly Meal Prep Plans" for your meal prep guide:

Planning your weekly meals in advance can save you time, money, and stress while helping you stay on track with your weight loss goals. Here are some meal prep plans to consider:

1. Basic Meal Prep Plan:

- **Breakfast:** Prepare a batch of overnight oats or Greek yogurt parfaits with berries for the week. Portion them into individual containers.
- **Lunch:** Make a large salad with lean protein (e.g., grilled chicken or tofu) and divide it into daily portions. Pack the dressing separately.
- **Dinner:** Cook a large batch of a balanced dinner recipe, such as baked salmon with veggies

or a quinoa and black bean bowl. Portion it into containers for the week.

2. Advanced Meal Prep Plan:

- **Breakfast:** Prepare a variety of breakfast options, such as egg muffins, smoothie packs (with pre-portioned ingredients), and chia seed pudding. Store them in the fridge or freezer.
- **Lunch:** Create a lunch menu with multiple options, like turkey and avocado wraps, lentil and vegetable soup, and quinoa salad. Make a different choice each day.
- **Dinner:** Plan out dinners for the week, including diverse recipes like veggie stir-fry, spaghetti squash with tomato and basil, and grilled chicken with lemon and herbs.

3. Vegetarian or Vegan Meal Prep Plan:

- **Breakfast:** Create plant-based breakfasts like tofu scramble with veggies, overnight chia oats, and avocado toast. Portion them into containers.
- **Lunch:** Focus on vegan lunches, such as chickpea salad wraps, lentil soup, and quinoa and roasted vegetable bowls.
- **Dinner:** Explore meatless dinners like stuffed bell peppers with rice and beans, sweet potato and black bean enchiladas, and vegetable curry.

4. Family Meal Prep Plan:

- **Breakfast:** Prep family-friendly options like whole-grain pancakes or waffles, yogurt parfaits, and oatmeal. Adjust portions to suit each family member.
- **Lunch:** Prepare lunches that can be customized, such as a sandwich or salad bar with various fillings and toppings. Let everyone assemble their lunch.
- **Dinner:** Cook large batches of family-favorite recipes like spaghetti with a choice of sauces, baked chicken with sides, and taco fixings for a build-your-own taco night.

5. Snack and Dessert Prep:

- **Snacks:** Create a snack drawer or shelf in your pantry and fridge with pre-portioned options like cut veggies with hummus, fruit cups, and portioned nuts or trail mix.
- **Desserts:** Have guilt-free dessert options ready, like chocolate avocado mousse, frozen banana "ice cream," or chia seed pudding.

6. Themed Cuisine Meal Prep Plan:

- Choose a different international cuisine theme each week, such as Mediterranean, Asian, or Mexican.
- Plan breakfast, lunch, and dinner recipes that fit the chosen cuisine theme, exploring different flavors and ingredients each week.

These weekly meal prep plans can be tailored to your dietary preferences, family size, and cooking skills. Having a clear plan and prepped meals on hand will make it easier to stick to your weight loss goals and maintain a healthy eating routine. In the following sections, we'll discuss long-term strategies for success and how to stay motivated on your journey.

CHAPTER ELEVEN

Staying Motivated

Absolutely! Here's a section on "Staying Motivated" for your meal prep guide:

Maintaining motivation on your weight loss journey can be challenging, but it's crucial for long-term success. Here are some strategies to help you stay motivated and committed to your goals.

1. Set Realistic and Achievable Goals:

- Start with small, achievable goals that you can track and celebrate. As you achieve these milestones, set new ones to keep yourself motivated.

2. Find Your Why:

- Identify the reasons why you want to lose weight and improve your health. This could be for physical better health, increased energy, improved self-confidence, or any other personal motivation. Remind yourself of your "why" regularly.

3. Visualize Your Success:

- Imagine yourself at your desired weight and fitness level. Visualizing your success can help reinforce your commitment to your goals.

4. Track Your Progress:

- Keep a record of your achievements, whether it's tracking your weight loss, measuring your fitness improvements, or documenting your healthier eating habits. Progress tracking can be a powerful motivator.

5. Reward Yourself:

- Celebrate your successes, big or small, with non-food rewards. Treat yourself to something special when you reach a milestone, like a new workout outfit or a spa day.

6. Surround Yourself with Support:

- Share your goals with friends and family who can provide encouragement and accountability.

Consider joining a weight loss support group or finding a workout buddy.

7. Keep It Fun:

- Find enjoyable ways to stay active. Whether it's dancing, hiking, or playing a sport you love, make exercise a fun part of your routine.

8. Mix Up Your Meals:

- Experiment with new recipes and flavors to keep your meals interesting. Trying new healthy foods can prevent mealtime boredom.

9. Embrace Setbacks as Learning Opportunities:

- If you have a setback or a day of indulgence, don't view it as failure. Instead, learn from it and use it as motivation to get back on track.

10. Stay Educated:

- Continuously educate yourself about nutrition, exercise, and healthy habits. The more you know, the better equipped you'll be to make informed choices.

11. Practice Self-Compassion:

- Be kind to yourself and avoid self-criticism. Weight loss journeys have ups and downs, and it's essential to be patient and forgiving with yourself.

12. Visual Reminders:

- Place visual reminders of your goals where you'll see them daily. This could be a motivational quote, a photo of a fitness role model, or an inspirational note to yourself.

13. Setbacks Are Not Failures:

- Remember that setbacks are a natural part of any journey, including weight loss. Don't be too hard on yourself if you slip up occasionally. What matters is your overall progress.

14. Seek Professional Guidance:

- If you're struggling with motivation or facing specific challenges, consider consulting a registered dietitian or a fitness trainer who can provide personalized guidance and support.

Staying motivated on your weight loss journey is a continuous process. By setting realistic goals, finding your personal motivation, tracking your progress, and embracing a positive mindset, you can maintain your motivation and work towards a healthier, happier you. In the final sections of this guide, we'll discuss strategies for handling setbacks and making your healthy lifestyle sustainable for the long term.

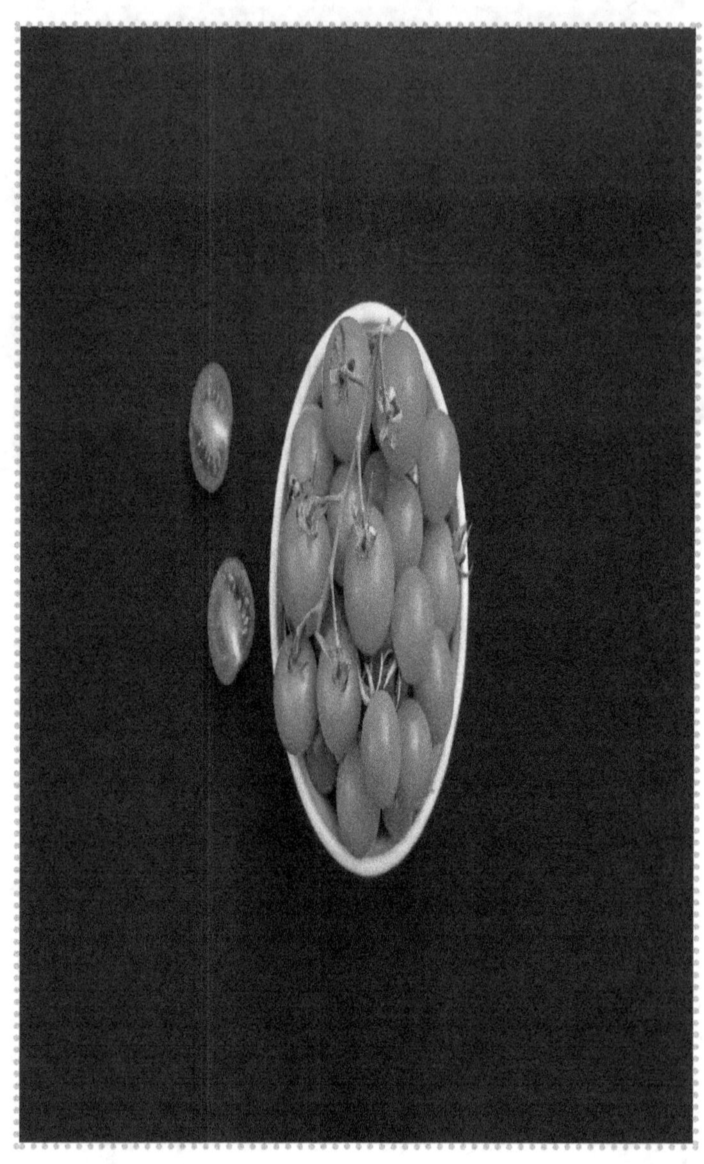

CHAPTER TWELVE

Maintaining a Healthy Lifestyle

Certainly! Here's a section on "Maintaining a Healthy Lifestyle" for your meal prep guide:

Achieving your weight loss goals is a significant accomplishment, but maintaining a healthy lifestyle over the long term is equally important. Here are some strategies to help you sustain your progress and enjoy a balanced, healthy life.

1. Build Sustainable Habits:

- Focus on building habits that you can maintain for life. Instead of thinking of your journey as a temporary diet, aim for lasting changes in your eating and exercise routines.

2. Practice Portion Control:

- Continue to be mindful of portion sizes, even after reaching your goal weight. This helps you maintain your desired weight and prevents overeating.

3. Stay Active:

- Exercise is an essential component of a healthy lifestyle. Find physical activities you enjoy and make them a regular part of your routine.

4. Listen to Your Body:

- Pay attention to your body's hunger and fullness cues. Eat when you're hungry and stop when you're satisfied.

5. Maintain a Balanced Diet:

- Continue to prioritize whole, nutrient-dense foods in your diet. Include a variety of fruits, vegetables, lean proteins, whole grains, and healthy fats in your meals.

6. Stay Hydrated:

- Drink plenty of water throughout the day to stay hydrated. Sometimes, thirst can be mistaken for hunger.

7. Plan Your Meals:

- Continue to plan and prep your meals in advance. Having healthy options readily available makes it easier to make nutritious choices.

8. Handle Setbacks Gracefully:

- Understand that setbacks are normal and part of life. When they occur, don't get discouraged; instead, use them as opportunities to learn and adjust.

9. Get Adequate Sleep:

- Prioritize quality sleep to support your overall health and well-being. Aim for 7-9 hours of sleep per night.

10. Manage Stress:

- Find healthy ways to manage stress, such as through meditation, yoga, or deep breathing exercises. Stress can impact your eating habits and overall health.

11. Stay Informed:

- Continue to educate yourself about nutrition and wellness. Stay up to date with reliable sources of information.

12. Regular Check-Ins:

- Schedule regular check-ins with yourself to evaluate your progress and make any necessary adjustments to your routine.

13. Seek Support:

- Stay connected with your support system, whether it's friends, family, or a support group. They can help you stay accountable and motivated.

14. Celebrate Success:

- Celebrate your achievements along the way. Recognize and reward yourself for reaching milestones and maintaining a healthy lifestyle.

15. Be Patient and Persistent:

- Remember that maintaining a healthy lifestyle is an ongoing journey. There will be ups and downs, but staying persistent and committed to your goals will help you succeed in the long run.

16. Set New Goals:

- Once you've achieved your initial weight loss goal, consider setting new health and fitness goals to keep yourself motivated and challenged.

Remember that maintaining a healthy lifestyle is about more than just the number on the scale. It's about feeling your best, having the energy to enjoy life, and reducing your risk of chronic diseases. By incorporating these strategies into your daily life, you can continue to thrive and enjoy the benefits of a balanced, healthy lifestyle for years to come.

In this guide, we've covered the fundamentals of meal prep, healthy recipes, snacks, desserts, and strategies for maintaining motivation and long-term success. Use this knowledge to create a plan that works for you and supports your health and wellness journey. Here's to your continued success and well-being!

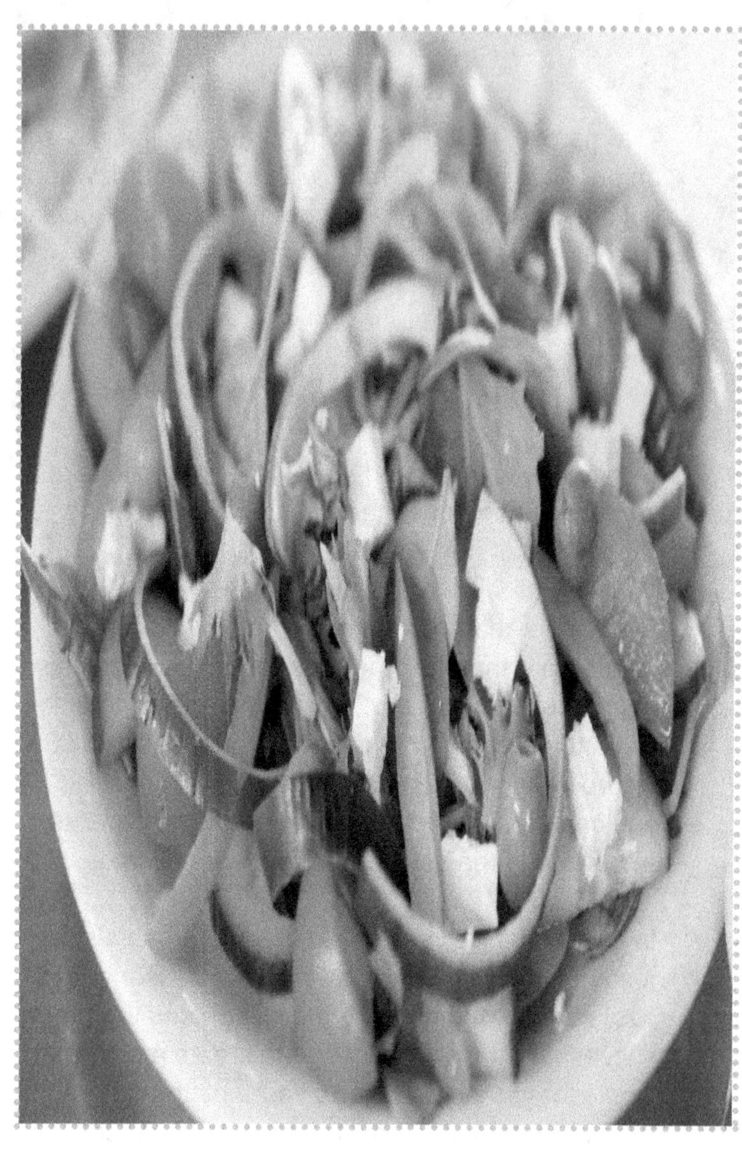

Conclusion

Congratulations on completing this comprehensive meal prep guide for weight loss! You've gained valuable insights into the world of meal preparation, nutritious recipes, and strategies for maintaining a healthy lifestyle. As you embark on your journey towards better health and weight management, remember that consistency and mindful choices are your allies.

In summary, here are the key takeaways from this guide:

- Meal prep is a powerful tool for achieving and maintaining your weight loss goals.
- Planning your meals in advance saves time, money, and helps you make healthier food choices.
- Healthy and delicious recipes can be the foundation of your meal prep routine, from breakfast to dinner and guilt-free dessert.
- Smart snacking can satisfy your cravings without derailing your progress.
- Staying motivated is essential for long-term success, and setting achievable goals and tracking your progress can keep you on course.
- The journey doesn't end with weight loss; maintaining a healthy lifestyle is about building sustainable habits, staying active, and practicing self-care.

Remember that your path to a healthier you is a personal one, and it's okay to tailor these strategies to fit your unique preferences and needs. Whether you're just beginning your journey or continuing to maintain your achievements, your commitment to a healthier lifestyle is commendable.

As you move forward, stay inspired, celebrate your successes, and be resilient in the face of challenges. You have the knowledge and tools to lead a happier, healthier life. Here's to your continued well-being and success!